Insulin Resistance Diet for Women Over 50

Dr. Christie Barron

D1533801

Disclaimer

Please keep in mind that the content in this book is solely for educational purposes. The information offered here is said to be reliable and trustworthy. The author makes no implication or intends to offer any warranty of accuracy for particular individual cases. Before beginning any diet or lifestyle habits, it is recommended that you contact a knowledgeable practitioner, such as your doctor. This book's material should not be utilized in place of expert counsel or professional guidance.

The author, publisher, and distributor expressly disclaim all liability, loss, damage, or danger incurred by persons who rely on the information in this book, whether directly or indirectly.

All intellectual property rights are retained. This book's information should not be replicated in any way, mechanically, electronically, photocopying, or by any other methods accessible

Table of Contents

Martha Jones's Success Story - How She Overcame Insulin Resistance

Martha Jones, 56, has been suffering from insulin resistance for a number of years. She'd been diagnosed with type 2 diabetes a few years before, and despite following her doctor's recommendations, she still suffered from high blood sugar levels and weight loss.

Martha had always been active and health-conscious, but as she aged, it became more difficult for her to maintain a healthy weight. She tried a variety of diets and workout regimes, but nothing worked. She felt upset and dismayed as if she were trapped in an endless cycle of weight increase and blood sugar rises.

Martha stumbled across an article regarding the link between insulin resistance and weight increase in women over the age of 50 one day. She was piqued and decided to conduct further study on the subject. She observed that insulin resistance is a prevalent issue among older women and that it can be a significant barrier to weight loss and good health.

Martha decided to act and began using some of the ideas she had learned. She began by altering her diet, focusing on meals strong in protein and fiber and low in carbs. She began eating more veggies, lean meats, and healthy fats while reducing her use of sugar and processed foods.

She also began exercising more often, including both cardio and weight training in her program. She discovered that exercising not only helped her lose weight but also helped her regulate her blood sugar levels and enhance her general health.

Martha's health improved significantly after a few months of implementing these new lifestyle adjustments. Her blood sugar levels were steady, and she was able to shed and maintain her weight loss. She felt better and had more energy than she had in years.

Martha's success story is frequent among women over the age of 50 who suffer from insulin resistance. They can overcome this disease and attain optimal health by making easy lifestyle adjustments such as modifying their diet and increasing their physical activity.

Insulin resistance develops when the cells of the body become less receptive to insulin, a hormone that regulates blood sugar levels. This can result in elevated blood sugar, weight gain, and other health issues. Insulin resistance is frequent in women over the age of 50, as their systems become less effective at digesting glucose and controlling insulin levels.

The good news is that insulin resistance may be controlled and even reversed by making modifications to one's diet and exercise routine. Women over 50 can regulate their blood sugar levels and reduce weight by eating a nutritious diet low in carbs and high in protein and fiber. They can also increase their insulin sensitivity and general health by including regular exercise in their lifestyle.

In conclusion, Martha's success story demonstrates that insulin resistance is not a death sentence and that modest lifestyle modifications may make a significant impact in treating this illness. Women over the age of 50 who suffer from insulin resistance should be inspired by Martha and take action to enhance their health and well-being.

Understanding Insulin Resistance

Insulin resistance occurs when the body's cells become less receptive to insulin, a pancreatic hormone that regulates blood sugar levels. This implies that the body is less able to absorb glucose, resulting in greater blood sugar levels and a variety of health issues.

What exactly is Insulin Resistance?
Insulin resistance is frequent in women over the age of 50, as their systems become less effective at digesting glucose and controlling insulin levels. This can result in a variety of health issues, such as type 2 diabetes, heart disease, and obesity.

Insulin resistance develops when the cells of the body become less sensitive to insulin. This means that the body must manufacture more insulin to maintain blood sugar levels. As the body struggles to keep up with the demands of insulin production, this can lead to a variety of health problems over time.

Causes of Insulin Resistance

A variety of variables can contribute to the development of insulin resistance. These are some examples:

Women over 50 are more likely to develop insulin resistance as their systems become less effective in processing glucose and regulating insulin levels.
Insulin resistance has a hereditary component, and some people are more prone to the illness than others.

A high-sugar, processed food, and unhealthy-fat diet can contribute to the development of insulin resistance.
A sedentary lifestyle can lead to insulin resistance, while frequent exercise improves insulin sensitivity.
Obesity: Excess body fat can interfere with insulin synthesis and control, increasing the risk of developing insulin resistance.

Insulin Resistance Symptoms

Insulin resistance is sometimes difficult to identify in its early stages since there are no visible signs. However, as the condition worsens, a variety of symptoms may appear, including:

High blood sugar levels: Insulin resistance can cause blood sugar levels to increase, resulting in a variety of health issues.

Weight gain: Insulin resistance can make losing weight difficult, if not impossible.

Weariness: As the body tries to metabolize glucose, insulin resistance can cause weariness and low energy levels.

Increased hunger: As the body tries to control blood sugar levels, insulin resistance can cause people to feel hungry more frequently.

Insulin resistance can cause excessive urine as the body attempts to remove excess glucose.

In conclusion, insulin resistance is a prevalent condition in women over the age of 50, and it can be caused by a variety of variables such as age, genetics, food, lack of exercise, and obesity. While there may be no obvious symptoms in the early stages, as the condition progresses, a variety of symptoms such as high blood sugar levels, weight gain, fatigue, increased hunger, and frequent urination may develop. Understanding the origins and symptoms of insulin resistance is the first step toward controlling the illness and improving general health and well-being.

The Importance of a Healthy Diet in Insulin Resistance

In women over 50, a nutritious diet is critical for treating insulin resistance. Women may control their blood sugar levels, lower insulin resistance, and enhance their general health and well-being by eating the correct foods and avoiding specific ones. In this chapter, we will address the importance of a balanced diet for insulin resistance, as well as offer advice for what to eat and avoid, as well as an example day's meal plan.

What to Eat and What Not to Eat

The key to treating insulin resistance is to consume a well-balanced diet rich in full, nutrient-dense foods. Women with insulin resistance should consume a diet high in fiber, protein, and healthy fats and low in sugar, processed carbs, and harmful fats. It is very critical to:

Avoid sugary meals and beverages: Sugary foods and beverages can raise blood sugar levels, worsening insulin resistance. Sugary foods, such as candy, soda, and baked goods, as well as foods containing added sugars, should be avoided by women who have insulin resistance.

Refined carbs, such as white bread, pasta, and rice, can also cause blood sugar levels to surge. Women with insulin resistance should avoid these items and instead choose whole-grain alternatives.

Choose good fats: Nuts, seeds, avocado, and fatty fish include healthy fats that can help increase insulin sensitivity. Women who have insulin resistance should eat these meals while avoiding harmful fats found in fried foods and processed snacks.

Consume plenty of fiber: Fiber is essential for controlling blood sugar levels and improving insulin sensitivity. Women who have insulin resistance should consume lots of fiber-rich meals such as fruits, vegetables, and whole grains.

Best Insulin Resistance Foods

In addition to avoiding particular meals, women with insulin resistance should incorporate a variety of foods in their diet. These are some examples:

Lean protein: Chicken, fish, tofu, and lentils are high in lean protein and can help manage blood sugar levels and increase insulin sensitivity.

Non-starchy veggies, such as broccoli, kale, spinach, and peppers, are low in calories and high in fiber, making them a perfect diet for insulin-resistant women.

Whole grains are high in fiber and can help manage blood sugar levels. Examples include brown rice, quinoa, and whole-grain bread.

As previously stated, healthy fats found in nuts, seeds, avocados, and fatty fish can help increase insulin sensitivity.

Exercise and Insulin Resistance

Exercise is critical in the control of insulin resistance in women over 50. Physical activity on a regular basis can help increase insulin sensitivity, lower blood sugar levels, and minimize the chance of developing diabetes and other chronic health disorders. In this chapter, we will explain the importance of exercise for insulin resistance, as well as present guidelines for different forms of exercise and a sample weekly exercise schedule.

The Value of Exercise

Exercise is an effective technique for controlling insulin resistance because it improves insulin sensitivity and glucose absorption in the body. It also aids in the reduction of inflammation and the reduction of blood pressure, both of which are linked to insulin resistance and other chronic health disorders.

Regular exercise has been demonstrated in studies to enhance insulin sensitivity and reduce blood sugar levels in women who are already insulin resistant. In fact, in certain circumstances, exercise has been demonstrated to be just as helpful as medicine in increasing insulin sensitivity.

Types of Insulin Resistance Exercise

There are several sorts of exercises that can help ladies with insulin resistance. These are some examples:

Aerobic activity, such as brisk walking, cycling, or swimming, can enhance insulin sensitivity and aid to reduce blood sugar levels. Most days of the week, aim for at least 30 minutes of moderate-intensity aerobic activity.

Resistance Training: Weightlifting and bodyweight workouts, for example, can assist to develop muscle mass and improve insulin sensitivity. Aim for two to three sessions of strength training per week.

High-Intensity Interval Training (HIIT): HIIT consists of brief bursts of intensive activity followed by rest intervals. Exercise of this nature has been demonstrated to enhance insulin sensitivity and reduce blood sugar levels. Aim for one to two high-intensity interval training sessions each week.

A Week's Worth of Exercise

Here's an example of a workout program designed specifically for ladies with insulin resistance:

- Monday: vigorous walking for 30 minutes
- Tuesday: Resistance exercise (squats, lunges, push-ups, etc.)
- Wednesday: 30 minutes of swimming or riding
- Thursday is a day of rest.
- Friday: High-intensity interval training (HIIT) (e.g., sprints, burpees, jumping jacks)
- Saturday: Resistance training (deadlifts, bench press, rowing, etc.)
- 30 minutes of vigorous walking on Sunday

It's vital to note that every woman's fitness regimen will be unique to her own demands and talents. If you are new to exercising or have any underlying health issues, talk with your healthcare physician before starting a new fitness program.

In conclusion, exercise is a crucial part of managing insulin resistance in women over 50. Aerobic exercise, strength training, and high-intensity interval training (HIIT) are all effective forms of exercise that can enhance insulin sensitivity and reduce blood sugar levels. Women can enhance their general health and well-being and lower their chance of acquiring diabetes and other chronic health disorders by including regular exercise in their routines.

Other Lifestyle Changes to Manage Insulin Resistance

While diet and exercise are important components in managing insulin resistance, women over 50 can make other lifestyle changes to help manage their condition. In this chapter, we'll talk about how to manage stress, get adequate sleep, and take supplements to treat insulin resistance.

Stress Administration

Although stress is an unavoidable part of life, chronic stress can impair insulin sensitivity and blood sugar levels. When the body is stressed, chemicals are released that might raise blood sugar levels and lead to insulin resistance. This is why it's critical for women over 50 to learn how to handle stress and limit its negative influence on their health.

Relaxation practices such as meditation, deep breathing, or yoga are helpful ways to handle stress. These techniques have been demonstrated to relieve stress and boost general well-being. Regular exercise, time spent in nature, and time spent with loved ones can all help to relieve stress.

The Value of Sleep

Getting adequate sleep is also essential for controlling insulin resistance. Sleep deprivation has been linked to decreased insulin sensitivity and an increased chance of developing diabetes. To support good sleep habits, aim for at least 7-8 hours of sleep every night and stick to a consistent sleep routine.

There are various tactics that might assist if you have difficulties sleeping, such as creating a calming sleep environment, avoiding electronic gadgets before night, and developing a regular sleep regimen.

Insulin Resistance Supplements

While a healthy diet and exercise are the most important factors in managing insulin resistance, there are a number of supplements that can help. Some of the most effective insulin resistance supplements are:

Omega-3 Fatty Acids: Omega-3 fatty acids have anti-inflammatory properties and can help increase insulin sensitivity. They may be found in fatty fish like salmon and tuna, as well as supplements.

Magnesium: Magnesium is an important mineral that helps with insulin sensitivity. It may be found in leafy greens, nuts, seeds, and as a supplement.

Chromium: Chromium is a mineral that can aid insulin sensitivity and blood sugar regulation. Whole grains, broccoli, and green beans, as well as supplements, contain it.

Vitamin D: Vitamin D helps with insulin sensitivity and may be gained from sun exposure, fortified meals, and supplements.

It is critical to highlight that supplements should not be utilized in place of a balanced diet and lifestyle. Before beginning any supplements, contact your healthcare physician to ensure that they are appropriate for you.

In conclusion, stress management, enough sleep, and supplement usage are further lifestyle adjustments that can aid in the management of insulin resistance in women over 50. Women may enhance their overall health and well-being and lower their chance of getting diabetes and other chronic health disorders by implementing these measures into their daily routines.

Insulin Resistance Monitoring and Management

Monitoring and controlling insulin resistance is a continuous process that demands focus and effort. In this chapter, we'll go through how to monitor insulin resistance, when to see a doctor and drugs that can help with insulin resistance management.

How to Track Insulin Resistance

Blood tests that detect glucose and insulin levels are the most frequent approach to assessing insulin resistance. These tests can be performed in a doctor's office or at home with the use of a glucose meter. It is critical to periodically measure blood sugar levels and keep track of the results in a journal or log.

Regular check-ups with a healthcare practitioner are another key strategy to manage insulin resistance. Your healthcare practitioner can check your general health and advise you on how to manage your insulin resistance during these sessions.

When Should You See a Doctor?

If you have indications of insulin resistance or are at risk of developing diabetes, you should consult a doctor. Insulin resistance symptoms include:

- Fatigue
- heightened thirst
- Urination on a regular basis
- Vision distortion
- Wounds that take a long time to heal

If you have a family history of diabetes or are overweight or obese, you may be at risk of developing insulin resistance and should visit your doctor on a frequent basis.

Insulin Resistance Treatments

Medication, in addition to lifestyle adjustments, can be used to address insulin resistance. Among the most often used insulin-resistance drugs are:

Metformin is a medicine that lowers blood sugar levels and improves insulin sensitivity. It is commonly taken for type 2 diabetes, although it can also be used to treat insulin resistance.

Thiazolidinediones are a kind of medicine that improves insulin sensitivity and decreases glucose synthesis in the liver. To control insulin resistance, they are frequently used in conjunction with other drugs.

GLP-1 Receptor Agonists: GLP-1 receptor agonists are a relatively new family of drugs that aid in blood sugar regulation by enhancing insulin secretion and decreasing glucose synthesis in the liver.

It's crucial to remember that drugs should only be used in conjunction with a healthy diet and lifestyle, and they should only be used with the supervision of a healthcare practitioner.

In conclusion, monitoring and controlling insulin resistance is a continuous process that demands attention and effort. Women over 50 can control their insulin resistance and lower their risk of developing diabetes and other chronic health disorders by consistently monitoring blood sugar levels, seeing a doctor for frequent check-ups, and using medicines as required.

BREAKFAST

Yogurt with berries and almonds from Greece

This high-protein breakfast is a delicious and nutritious way to start your day. Creamy Greek yogurt, antioxidant-rich berries, and crunchy almonds will satisfy your hunger and keep you satisfied until lunch.

Time allotted: 5 minutes

1 serving

Ingredients:
1 cup plain Greek yogurt
1/2 cup berries, mixed
1 tbsp. sliced almonds

Directions:
Add Greek yogurt to a bowl and top with mixed berries and chopped almonds.
Serve immediately and enjoy.

Information about nutrition:
220 calories
21g protein
Fat: 7g
21g carbohydrate

4g fiber

Oatmeal with cinnamon and walnuts

This substantial cup of oats is ideal for chilly mornings. The fiber-rich oats, heart-healthy walnuts, and metabolism-boosting cinnamon make it an ideal breakfast meal for weight reduction and belly fat.

Time allotted: 10 minutes

1 serving

Ingredients:

1/2 cup oats, rolled

1 cup of water

1 tbsp. chopped walnuts

1/2 teaspoon cinnamon powder

Directions:

Bring a small saucepan of water to a boil. Reduce the heat to low and add the rolled oats. Simmer for 5-7 minutes, or until the oats are tender and the liquid has been absorbed.

Sprinkle the oats with chopped walnuts and cinnamon.

Serve immediately and enjoy.

Information about nutrition:
280 calories

9g protein

Fat: 11g

38g carbohydrate

7g fiber

Omelette with vegetables and avocado slices

This protein-rich omelet is an excellent breakfast option for losing weight and abdominal fat. All morning long, the mix of eggs, veggies, and healthy fats will keep you full and content.

Time allotted: 15 minutes

1 serving

Ingredients:
2 eggs

1/4 cup chopped bell pepper

1/4 cup chopped onion

1/4 cup chopped mushroom

1/2 sliced avocado

Season with salt and pepper to taste.

1 tablespoon of olive oil

Directions:

Whisk together the eggs, salt, and pepper in a small bowl.

In a nonstick skillet over medium heat, heat the olive oil. Sauté the diced veggies for 3-4 minutes, or until tender.

Cook for 2-3 minutes, or until the bottom is set, with the egg mixture. Cook for another minute after flipping the omelet.

Place the omelet on a platter and garnish with avocado slices.

Serve immediately and enjoy.

Information about nutrition:

320 calories

16g protein

Fat: 23g

13g carbohydrate

7g fiber

Quinoa porridge with fruit and almond milk

This gluten-free and dairy-free quinoa porridge is an excellent breakfast option for losing weight and abdominal fat. It's high in protein and fiber, and with the addition of

almond milk and berries, it's a delightful and nutritious breakfast alternative.
Time allotted: 20 minutes
1 serving

Ingredients:
1/2 cup washed quinoa
1 cup almond milk, unsweetened
1/2 cup berries, mixed
1 teaspoon honey
1/4 teaspoon cinnamon powder

Directions:
Combine the quinoa and almond milk in a small saucepan. Bring to a boil, then lower to low heat and continue to cook for 15-20 minutes, or until the quinoa is tender and the mixture is thick and creamy.
Mix in the honey and cinnamon powder.
Garnish with mixed berries.
Serve immediately and enjoy.

Information about nutrition:
300 calories
10g protein
Fat: 7g
50g carbohydrates

7g fiber

Sweet potato toast with almond butter and banana slices

This gluten-free and vegan breakfast meal is a healthier alternative to bread. Sweet potato slices are roasted till crispy and then topped with creamy almond butter and sliced banana, making it an ideal weight reduction and belly fat breakfast alternative.

Time allotted: 30 minutes

1 serving

Ingredients:

1 medium sweet potato, cut into

1/4-inch thick slices lengthwise

two tbsp almond butter

1/4 teaspoon ground cinnamon

1/2 medium banana, cut

Directions:

Preheat the oven to 400 degrees Fahrenheit.

Using parchment paper, line a baking sheet.

Place the sweet potato slices on a baking pan and bake for 20-25 minutes or until soft and crispy around the edges.

Remove from oven and set aside for a few minutes to cool.

Top each sweet potato slice with almond butter.

Sprinkle with ground cinnamon and top with sliced banana.

Serve immediately and enjoy.

Information about nutrition:
280 calories
7g protein
Fat: 13g
36g carbohydrate
7g fiber

Cottage cheese topped with sliced peaches and cinnamon

This high-protein, low-calorie breakfast meal is ideal for losing weight and abdominal fat. A tasty and nutritious breakfast alternative, cottage cheese is topped with luscious peaches and a touch of cinnamon.

Time allotted: 5 minutes
1 serving

Ingredients:
1/2 cup cottage cheese (low-fat)

1 medium-sliced peach
1/4 teaspoon cinnamon powder

Directions:
Place cottage cheese in a mixing basin.
Sprinkle with ground cinnamon and top with sliced peaches.
Serve immediately and enjoy.

Information about nutrition:
140 calories
15g protein
Fat: 2g
18g carbohydrate
2g fiber

Chia seed pudding with coconut milk and fruit of various colors

This vegan and gluten-free chia seed pudding is an excellent breakfast option for losing weight and belly fat. Chia seeds are combined with coconut milk and topped with mixed berries to create a nutritious and tasty breakfast alternative.

Total time: 5 minutes (plus 2 hours for cooling)
1 serving

Ingredients:
1 tablespoon chia seeds
1 cup coconut milk, unsweetened
1/2 cup berries, mixed
1 tbsp. honey (optional)

Directions:
Chia seeds and coconut milk should be combined in a dish. To blend, stir everything together thoroughly.
Refrigerate for at least 2 hours or overnight, or until the liquid thickens and the chia seeds are completely hydrated.
If desired, top with mixed berries and sprinkle with honey.
Serve immediately and enjoy.

Information about nutrition:
330 calories
7g protein
Fat: 23g
24g carbohydrate
14g dietary fiber

Eggs scrambled with spinach and feta cheese

This protein-rich breakfast meal is ideal for losing weight and abdominal fat. Scrambled eggs, sautéed spinach, and crumbled feta cheese combine to provide a delectable and healthy meal that will keep you full and content.

Time allotted: 10 minutes

1 serving

Ingredients:

two huge eggs

1 cup fresh baby spinach

1/4 cup feta cheese, crumbled

1 tablespoon extra virgin olive oil

Season with salt and pepper to taste.

Directions:

Whisk together eggs and a touch of salt and pepper in a mixing basin.

In a nonstick skillet over medium-high heat, heat the olive oil.

Cook until the baby spinach is wilted, about 1-2 minutes.

Pour in the whisked eggs and scramble for 3-4 minutes, or until cooked through.

Cook for a further 1-2 minutes, or until the feta cheese melts, over the eggs.
Serve immediately and enjoy.

Information about nutrition:
350 calories
22g protein
Fat: 26g
4g carbohydrate
1g fiber

Smashed avocado on whole grain bread with cured salmon

This breakfast meal is a nutritious and tasty way to start the day. Smashed avocado and smoked salmon are spread over whole-grain bread for a protein-packed breakfast that will leave you full and happy.
Time allotted: 10 minutes
1 serving

Ingredients:
2 healthy grain bread pieces, toasted
1/2 avocado, mashed 2 ounces cured salmon
Season with salt and pepper to taste.

Directions:

Toast the pieces of bread.

Spread smashed avocado on each slice of bread equally.

Sprinkle with salt and pepper and top with smoked salmon.

Serve immediately and enjoy.

Information about nutrition:

350 calories

22g protein

Fat: 21g

23g carbohydrate

8g fiber

Spinach, banana, almond milk, and protein powder smoothie bowl

This morning smoothie bowl is ideal for losing weight and abdominal fat. It's created with spinach, banana, almond milk, and protein powder, so it's a high-protein, nutrient-dense meal that'll keep you full and content.

Time allotted: 5 minutes

1 serving

Ingredients:

1 frozen banana

1 cup fresh baby spinach
1/2 cup almond milk, unsweetened
1 scoop protein powder vanilla
1 tbsp. almond butter
Toppings include sliced bananas, chia seeds, and sliced almonds.

Directions:
Blend a frozen banana, baby spinach, almond milk, protein powder, and almond butter in a blender.
Blend until the mixture is smooth and creamy.
Fill a bowl halfway with the smoothie.
Top with banana slices, chia seeds, and almond slices.
Serve immediately and enjoy.

Information about nutrition:
360 calories
25g protein
Fat: 14g
43g carbohydrate
10g dietary fiber

LUNCH

Chicken Breast Grilled with Roasted Vegetables

This is a traditional weight-loss recipe. Grilled chicken breast is high in protein and low in calories, while roasted veggies add fiber and minerals. This meal takes 30 minutes to prepare and serves 4 people.

Ingredients:
4 breasts of chicken
2 cups mixed veggies (broccoli, bell peppers, onions, zucchini, for example)
2 tablespoons olive oil
1 teaspoon garlic powder
1 teaspoon paprika
Season with salt and pepper to taste.

Directions:
Preheat the grill to medium-high temperature. Garlic powder, paprika, salt, and pepper season the chicken breasts.
Grill the chicken for 5-7 minutes per side, or until done.
Toss the veggies in a bowl with olive oil, salt, and pepper.

Roast the veggies for 15-20 minutes at 400°F, or until tender.
Grilled chicken should be served with roasted veggies.

Nutrition facts (per serving):
240 calories
30g protein
Fat: 9g
11g carbohydrate
4g fiber

Salad of mixed greens with grilled salmon and avocado

The grilled salmon and avocado provide healthful fats and protein to this salad. The mixed greens contain fiber as well as other important elements. This meal takes 20 minutes to prepare and serves 2 people.

Ingredients:
2 fillets of salmon
4 cups greens, mixed
1 sliced avocado
1/4 cup red onion, sliced
2 tablespoons olive oil
2 tablespoons lemon juice

Season with salt and pepper to taste.

Directions:
Preheat the grill to medium-high temperature.
Season both sides of the salmon fillets with salt and pepper.
Grill the salmon for 4-5 minutes per side, or until done.
Toss the mixed greens, avocado, and red onion with olive oil, lemon juice, salt, and pepper in a large mixing bowl.
Serve the salad on two dishes, topped with the grilled salmon.

Nutrition facts (per serving):
450 calories
34g protein
Fat: 30g
14g carbohydrate
9g fiber

Chili with Turkey and Mixed Vegetables

This turkey chili is high in protein and fiber thanks to the turkey and mixed veggies. This meal takes 40 minutes to prepare and serves 6 people.

Ingredients:
1 pound ground turkey
1 can drained and rinsed black beans
1 tomato can, diced
2 cups mixed veggies (for example, bell peppers, onions, and zucchini)
2 minced garlic cloves
1 tablespoon olive oil
1 teaspoon chili powder
1 teaspoon cumin
Season with salt and pepper to taste.

Directions:
In a large saucepan, heat the olive oil over medium-high heat.
Cook until the ground turkey is browned, breaking it up into tiny pieces with a wooden spoon.
Cook for 5-7 minutes, or until the mixed veggies and garlic are soft.
To the saucepan, add the chopped tomatoes, black beans, chili powder, cumin, salt, and pepper.
Cook the chili for 20-25 minutes at a low heat.
Serve the chili immediately.

Nutrition facts (per serving):
250 calories
22g protein
Fat: 9g
23g carbohydrate
7g fiber

Salad with Tuna, Lettuce Cups, and Cherry Tomatoes

This tuna salad is a light and refreshing lunch choice that is strong in protein and low in calories. By serving it in lettuce cups instead of bread or crackers, you may cut back on your total calorie consumption. This meal takes 10 minutes to prepare and serves 2 people.

Ingredients:
2 drained tuna cans
1/4 cup celery diced
1/4 cup red onion diced
2 tablespoons plain Greek yogurt
1 tablespoon Dijon mustard
1 tablespoon lemon juice
Season with salt and pepper to taste.
8 to ten lettuce leaves
1 cup halved cherry tomatoes

Directions:
Combine the tuna, celery, red onion, Greek yogurt, Dijon mustard, lemon juice, salt, and pepper in a large mixing bowl.
Distribute the tuna salad among the lettuce cups.
Serve the lettuce cups alongside cherry tomatoes.

Nutrition facts (per serving):
200 calories
30g protein
Fat: 4g
9g Carbohydrates
3g fiber

Wrapped Veggies with Hummus and Sprouts

This vegetarian wrap is a substantial and fulfilling lunch choice that is high in fiber and minerals thanks to the veggies and hummus. This meal takes 15 minutes to prepare and serves 2 people.

Ingredients:
2 whole grain tortillas
1 hummus cup

1/2 cup carrots, shredded
1/2 cup red cabbage, shredded
a half-cup sprouts
1/4 cup red onion, sliced
Season with salt and pepper to taste.

Directions:
Distribute the hummus equally among the tortillas.
Divide the tortillas with the shredded carrots, red cabbage, sprouts, and red onion.
Season to taste with salt and pepper.
Roll the tortillas tightly and cut them in half.

Nutrition facts (per serving):
300 calories
10g protein
Fat: 12g
39g carbohydrate
10g dietary fiber

Soup with Lentils and Mixed Vegetables

This lentil soup is a substantial and hearty meal that is packed with protein and fiber. The mixed veggies provide additional nutrition and taste. This meal takes 45 minutes to prepare and serves 6 people.

Ingredients:
1 cup green lentils, dry
1 diced onion
2 minced garlic cloves
2 cups mixed veggies (carrots, celery, zucchini, etc.)
1 tomato can, diced
6 cups vegetable broth (low sodium)
1 teaspoon dried thyme
Season with salt and pepper to taste.

Directions:
Rinse the lentils well and remove any trash or stones.
Heat the chopped onion and garlic in a large saucepan over medium-high heat. Cook until the onion has become transparent.
Cook for 5-7 minutes, or until the veggies are soft.
To the saucepan, add the lentils, chopped tomatoes, vegetable broth, dried thyme, salt, and pepper.
Bring the soup to a boil, then lower to a simmer.

Cook until the lentils are cooked, about 30-35 minutes.
Serve the soup immediately.

Nutrition facts (per serving):
200 calories
14g protein
Fat: 1g
36g carbohydrate
12g dietary fiber

Grilled Portobello Mushroom Salad with Quinoa

This quinoa salad with grilled portobello mushrooms is a wonderful and healthful vegetarian lunch alternative. The portobello mushroom makes an excellent meat alternative, and the quinoa salad provides protein and fiber. This meal takes 30 minutes to prepare and serves 2 people.

Ingredients:
2 portobello mushroom caps, big
2 tablespoons balsamic vinegar
2 tablespoons olive oil
Season with salt and pepper to taste.
1 cup quinoa, cooked

1/2 cup cucumber, diced
1/2 cup red bell pepper, chopped
1/4 cup fresh parsley, chopped
2 tablespoons lemon juice
1 tablespoon olive oil

Directions:
Preheat the grill to medium-high temperature.
Whisk together the balsamic vinegar, olive oil, salt, and pepper in a small basin.
Brush the balsamic mixture over the portobello mushroom caps.
Grill the mushrooms for 5-7 minutes per side, or until they are soft.
Combine the cooked quinoa, diced cucumber, diced red bell pepper, chopped parsley, lemon juice, olive oil, salt, and pepper in a large mixing bowl.
Serve the quinoa salad beside the grilled portobello mushrooms.

Nutrition facts (per serving):
250 calories
9g protein
Fat: 12g
28g carbohydrate
6g fiber

Salmon Baked with Roasted Asparagus

This baked salmon with roasted asparagus is a filling and healthful lunch choice. This meal takes 30 minutes to prepare and serves 2 people.

Ingredients:

2 fillets of salmon
2 tablespoons olive oil
Season with salt and pepper to taste.
1 pound trimmed asparagus 1 lemon, sliced

Directions:

Preheat the oven to 400 degrees Fahrenheit.
Line a baking sheet with parchment paper and place the salmon fillets on it.
Season the salmon fillets with salt and pepper after brushing them with olive oil.
Brush the asparagus with olive oil and arrange it over the salmon fillets.
Serve the salmon fillets with lemon slices on top.
Bake for 12-15 minutes, or until the salmon is well cooked and the asparagus is soft.
Serve immediately.

Nutrition facts (per serving):
300 calories
30g protein
Fat: 18g
8g carbohydrate
4g fiber

Stir-Fry Chicken with Mixed Vegetables and Brown Rice

This chicken stir-fry with mixed veggies and brown rice is a quick and simple protein and fiber-rich lunch choice. This meal takes 20 minutes to prepare and serves 2 people.

Ingredients:
1 cup brown rice, cooked
2 sliced chicken breasts
2 tbsp olive oil
Season with salt and pepper to taste.
1 sliced red bell pepper
1 sliced zucchini
1 cup sliced mushrooms
1 minced garlic clove
1 tablespoon soy sauce
1 teaspoon sesame oil

Directions:

Heat the olive oil in a large pan over medium-high heat.

Season the chicken slices with salt & pepper and place them in the skillet. Cook for 5-7 minutes, or until both sides are browned.

To the skillet, add the sliced bell pepper, zucchini, mushrooms, and minced garlic. Cook for 5-7 minutes longer, or until the veggies are soft.

In the skillet, combine the cooked brown rice, soy sauce, and sesame oil. Cook for another 1-2 minutes, or until heated through, stirring constantly.

Serve immediately.

Nutrition facts (per serving):

400 calories

35g protein

Fat: 14g

34g carbohydrate

6g fiber

Quinoa Bowl with Roasted Vegetables, Avocado, and Mixed Greens

This delicious and healthful quinoa meal with mixed greens, roasted veggies, and avocado is strong in protein and fiber. This meal takes 40 minutes to prepare and serves two people.

Ingredients:

1 cup quinoa, cooked
4 cups greens, mixed
1 small peeled and sliced sweet potato
1 small sliced red onion
1 sliced red bell pepper
1 tbsp olive oil
Season with salt and pepper to taste.
1 avocado, sliced
2 tablespoons lemon juice

Directions:

Preheat the oven to 400 degrees Fahrenheit.
On a baking sheet lined with parchment paper, place the diced sweet potato, sliced red onion, and sliced red bell pepper.
Season with salt and pepper and drizzle with olive oil.

Roast for 20-25 minutes, or until soft and browned in the oven.

Combine the cooked quinoa, mixed greens, avocado slices, and lemon juice in a large mixing basin.

Serve the quinoa and greens combination with the roasted veggies on top.

Nutrition facts (per serving):
400 calories
10g protein
Fat: 22g
45g carbohydrate
14g dietary fiber

DINNER

Steamed Broccoli and Cauliflower with Grilled Chicken Breast

This recipe is ideal for individuals who wish to eat healthy while yet enjoying a tasty supper. Grilled chicken breast is a lean protein source that will keep you full and happy, while steamed broccoli and cauliflower are high in vitamins and fiber.

Time allotted: 30 minutes

Servings per recipe: 4

Ingredients:
4 skinless, boneless chicken breasts
2 cups florets broccoli
2 cups florets cauliflower
1 tablespoon extra virgin olive oil
Season with salt and pepper to taste.

Directions:
Preheat the grill to medium-high.
Season the chicken breasts with salt and pepper after rubbing them with olive oil.
Grill the chicken for 6-8 minutes per side, or until done.
Steam broccoli and cauliflower for 8-10 minutes, or until soft, while the chicken is cooking.
Chicken should be served with steamed broccoli and cauliflower.

Per serving nutritional information:
220 calories
32g protein
Fat: 7g
8g carbohydrate
4g fiber

Salmon Baked with Roasted Brussels Sprouts

Salmon is high in omega-3 fatty acids, which can help to decrease inflammation and enhance heart health. This recipe is high in vitamins and antioxidants since it is served with roasted Brussels sprouts.

Time allotted: 35 minutes

Servings per recipe: 4

Ingredients:

4 fillets of salmon

1 pound trimmed and halved Brussels sprouts

2 tbsp of olive oil

Season with salt and pepper to taste.

Directions:

Preheat the oven to 400 degrees Fahrenheit.

Using parchment paper, line a baking sheet.

Place the salmon fillets and Brussels sprouts on a baking pan and set aside.

Season with salt and pepper and drizzle with olive oil.

Bake for 20-25 minutes, or until the salmon is done and the Brussels sprouts are soft.

Per serving nutritional information:
300 calories
27g protein
Fat: 19g
9g Carbohydrates
4g fiber

Meatballs of Turkey with Zucchini Noodles and Tomato Sauce

Using zucchini noodles instead of regular spaghetti is an excellent method to reduce carbohydrates and calories. This meal is a wonderful and nutritious alternative to spaghetti and meatballs when paired with turkey meatballs and tomato sauce.
Time allotted: 40 minutes
Servings per recipe: 4

Ingredients:
1 pound turkey ground
1 pound almond flour
1 egg
2 minced garlic cloves
1 tsp. dried oregano
1 teaspoon of salt
4 spiralized medium zucchini
1 can (14.5 oz) chopped tomatoes

1 tablespoon extra virgin olive oil
Season with salt and pepper to taste.

Directions:
Preheat the oven to 400 degrees Fahrenheit.
Combine ground turkey, almond flour, egg, garlic, oregano, and salt in a large mixing bowl.
Place the meatball mixture on a baking sheet and shape it into 16 meatballs.
Bake the meatballs for 20-25 minutes, or until done.
In a large pan over medium heat, heat the olive oil while the meatballs are cooking.
Sauté the spiralized zucchini for 2-3 minutes, or until soft.
Cook for 5-10 minutes, or until the chopped tomatoes are cooked through.
Serve meatballs with tomato sauce on top of zucchini noodles.

Per serving nutritional information:
290 calories
27g protein
Fat: 17g
11g carbohydrate
4g fiber

Stir-Fried Beef with Mixed Vegetables and Brown Rice

The lean meat and varied veggies in this beef stir-fry are high in protein and fiber. This recipe is satisfying and healthful when served over brown rice.

Time allotted: 30 minutes

Servings per recipe: 4

Ingredients:

1 pound flank steak, thinly sliced

2 cups mixed veggies (bell peppers, broccoli, snow peas, etc.)

2 minced garlic cloves

1 tablespoon extra virgin olive oil

1 teaspoon of soy sauce

Season with salt and pepper to taste.

2 cups brown rice, cooked

Directions:

In a large pan over high heat, heat the olive oil.

Stir-fry the sliced meat and garlic in the pan for 2-3 minutes, or until browned.

Continue to stir-fry the veggies in the pan for 3-4 minutes, or until they are tender-crisp.

Season with salt and pepper after adding the soy sauce.
Serve the beef stir-fry over brown rice.

Per serving nutritional information:
350 calories
26g protein
Fat: 11g
40g carbohydrates
6g fiber

Shrimp grilled with roasted peppers and onions

This grilled shrimp meal is low in calories and high in protein, making it an excellent choice for dieters. Roasted peppers and onions enhance the flavor and nutrients of the dish.
Time allotted: 25 minutes
Servings per recipe: 4

Ingredients:
1 pound big peeled and deveined shrimp
2 sliced bell peppers 1 sliced onion 2 teaspoons olive oil
Season with salt and pepper to taste.

Directions:

Preheat the grill to medium-high.

Thread the shrimp onto the skewers.

Season the sliced peppers and onions with salt and pepper after tossing them in olive oil.

Grill the shrimp and veggies for 2-3 minutes per side, or until the shrimp are pink and the vegetables are soft.

Grilled shrimp should be served with roasted peppers and onions.

Per serving nutritional information:

180 calories

25g protein

Fat: 8g

6g carbohydrate

2g fiber

Cauliflower Rice with Chicken Curry

Cauliflower rice, rather than conventional rice, is an excellent method to reduce calories and carbohydrates. This recipe is a nutritious and filling supper when paired with tasty chicken curry.

Time allotted: 35 minutes

Servings per recipe: 4

Ingredients:

1 pound boneless, skinless chicken breasts, sliced

1 tablespoon extra virgin olive oil

1 diced onion

2 minced garlic cloves

1 teaspoon curry powder

1 (14.5 oz) can of chopped tomatoes

1 can (13.5 oz) coconut cream

1 cauliflower head, shredded into "rice"

Season with salt and pepper to taste.

Directions:

In a large pan over medium heat, heat the olive oil.

Sauté the chicken, onion, and garlic in the pan for 5-7 minutes, or until the chicken is browned.

Cook for another minute after adding the curry powder.

Bring the diced tomatoes and coconut milk to a simmer in the pan.

Simmer for 10-15 minutes, or until the chicken is done and the sauce has thickened.

Meanwhile, in a separate pan, heat the oil over medium-high heat.

Cook for 3-4 minutes, or until the cauliflower rice is cooked, in the skillet.

Season the cauliflower rice with salt and pepper to taste.

Serve with cauliflower rice and chicken curry.

Per serving nutritional information:
320 calories
25g protein
Fat: 18g
15g carbohydrate
5g fiber

Sweet Potato Bake with Black Bean Chili

The black bean chili and sweet potato in this vegetarian recipe are high in fiber and protein. For those aiming to reduce weight, it's a satisfying and healthful supper option.

Time allotted: 1 hour
Servings per recipe: 4

Ingredients:
4 large sweet potatoes
1 (14.5 oz) can of chopped tomatoes
1 can (15 oz) washed and drained black beans
1 bell pepper, diced

1 onion, diced
2 garlic cloves, minced
1 teaspoon of chili powder
1 tablespoon extra virgin olive oil
Season with salt and pepper to taste.

Directions:
Preheat the oven to 400 degrees Fahrenheit (200 degrees Celsius).

Clean the sweet potatoes and puncture them with a fork.

Bake the sweet potatoes on a baking pan for 45-50 minutes, or until cooked.

Meanwhile, in a large pan over medium heat, heat the olive oil.

Sauté the diced bell pepper, onion, and garlic in the pan for 5-7 minutes, or until the veggies are soft.

Add the chili powder, chopped tomatoes, and black beans, and mix well.

Simmer for 10-15 minutes, or until the chili thickens.

Season with salt and pepper to taste.

Serve with roasted sweet potatoes and black bean chili.

Per serving nutritional information:
350 calories
10g protein
Fat: 6g
68g carbohydrate
16g dietary fiber

Chicken grilled with quinoa salad and mixed vegetables

This grilled chicken entrée is accompanied by a nutritious quinoa salad and mixed veggies, making it a well-balanced and nutritious lunch.
Time allotted: 35 minutes
Servings per recipe: 4

Ingredients:
1 pound skinless boneless chicken breasts
2 cups quinoa, cooked
2 cups mixed veggies (zucchini, bell peppers, cherry tomatoes, etc.)
2 tbsp of olive oil
two tbsp balsamic vinegar
Season with salt and pepper to taste.

Directions:
Preheat the grill to medium-high.

Season the chicken with salt and pepper after brushing it with olive oil.
Grill the chicken for 5-6 minutes per side, or until done.
Meanwhile, in a separate pan, heat the oil over medium-high heat.
Sauté the mixed veggies in the pan for 3-4 minutes, or until tender-crisp.
To prepare a dressing, mix together olive oil and balsamic vinegar in a small bowl.
Toss the cooked quinoa and mixed veggies with the dressing in a large mixing basin.
Grilled chicken should be served with quinoa salad and mixed veggies.

Per serving nutritional information:
340 calories
30g protein
Fat: 14g
24g carbohydrate
5g fiber

Beef Kebab with a Variety of Grilled Vegetables

For a nutritious and savory lunch, mix these beef kebabs with grilled veggies. Serve over brown rice for a full and well-balanced dinner.

Time allotted: 30 minutes
Servings per recipe: 4

Ingredients:
1 pound sliced into 1-inch pieces beef sirloin
2 bell peppers, peeled and sliced into 1-inch pieces
1 red onion, peeled and sliced into 1-inch pieces
1 zucchini (cut into rounds)
2 tbsp of olive oil
two tbsp balsamic vinegar
2 minced garlic cloves
Season with salt and pepper to taste.

Directions:
Preheat the grill to medium-high.
Thread beef cubes onto skewers, alternately with bell pepper, red onion, and zucchini slices.
Season the skewers with salt and pepper after brushing them with olive oil.
Grill the skewers for 8-10 minutes, flipping regularly, or until the meat is cooked to your liking.

Meanwhile, make the dressing by whisking together the olive oil, balsamic vinegar, and minced garlic in a small bowl.

Brush the dressing over the mixed veggies.

Grill the veggies for 3-4 minutes per side, or until they are tender-crisp.

Serve the meat kebabs with grilled veggies.

Per serving nutritional information:
280 calories
24g protein
Fat: 14g
14g carbohydrate
3g fiber

Tuna Steak Grilled with Roasted Sweet Potato and Mixed Greens

For a healthful and filling meal, serve this grilled tuna steak with roasted sweet potato and mixed greens.

Time allotted: 40 minutes
Servings per recipe: 4

Ingredients:
four tuna steaks
2 peeled and cut into 1-inch pieces sweet potatoes

4 cups greens, mixed
2 tbsp of olive oil
1 teaspoon honey
1 tbsp. Dijon mustard
Season with salt and pepper to taste.

Directions:

Preheat the grill to medium-high.
Season tuna steaks with salt and pepper after brushing with olive oil.
Grill tuna steaks for 2-3 minutes per side, or until done to preference.
Preheat the oven to 400°F (200°C) in the meantime.
Season the sweet potato cubes with salt and pepper after tossing them with 1 tablespoon of olive oil.
Bake sweet potatoes for 20-25 minutes, or until cooked.
To prepare a dressing, mix together the remaining olive oil, honey, and Dijon mustard in a small bowl.
Mix the dressing into the mixed greens.
Grilled tuna steak should be served with roasted sweet potato and mixed greens.

Per serving nutritional information:
300 calories
28g protein
Fat: 10g
24g carbohydrate
4g fiber

SNACK

Almond butter with apple slices

Introduction: This snack is both sweet and filling. The almond butter delivers protein and healthy fats, while the apple gives fiber and minerals.
Time allotted: 5 minutes

Ingredients:
1 apple, sliced
two tbsp almond butter
Cut the apple into slices.
On the slices, spread the almond butter.

Nutritional data (per serving):
206 calories
Fat: 11g
26g carbohydrate
5g fiber

5g protein

Hummus with raw vegetables

This snack is ideal for individuals who enjoy crisp and fresh veggies. Hummus contains protein and healthy fats, which help you feel filled for longer.

Time allotted: 10 minutes
Servings per recipe: 2

Ingredients:
1 cup washed and drained canned chickpeas
2 tablespoons tahini
2 minced garlic cloves
2 tablespoons lemon juice
1/4 teaspoon salt
1/4 cup of water
Raw veggies (carrot sticks, celery sticks, cucumber slices, and bell pepper strips, for example)

Directions:
Combine the chickpeas, tahini, minced garlic, lemon juice, and salt in a food processor.
Pulse the mixture until it reaches the consistency of a smooth paste.

Slowly add water to the food processor while it is running until the hummus achieves the appropriate consistency.

Serve the hummus in a serving dish with different raw veggies for dipping.

Per serving nutritional information:
150 calories
Fat: 7g
16g carbohydrate
7g protein

Hard-boiled egg with cucumber slices

This snack is simple but filling. Cucumbers give a pleasant crunch and water, while hard-boiled eggs deliver protein.

Time allotted: 15 minutes

Ingredients:
1 hard-boiled egg
1/2 sliced cucumber

Directions:
Peel the hard-boiled egg.
Cut the cucumber into slices.
Serve as a group.

Nutritional data (per serving):
99 calories
Fat: 5g
5g carbohydrate
1g fiber
8g protein

Nuts and seeds mixed

This snack is ideal for individuals looking for something flavorful and crispy. Nuts and seeds provide healthy fats, protein, and fiber, which can make you feel full and content.
Time allotted: 5 minutes
1 serving = 1/4 cup mixed nuts and seeds (almonds, walnuts, cashews, pumpkin seeds, sunflower seeds, etc.)

Step 1: Measure out the mixed nuts and seeds.
Serve as a snack.

Nutritional data (per serving):
196 calories
Fat: 16g
6g carbohydrate
3g fiber
8g protein

Paprika-roasted chickpeas

This snack is a more nutritious alternative to potato chips. Chickpeas are high in protein and fiber, and paprika provides a smoky, flavorful taste.

Time allotted: 40 minutes
Servings per recipe: 4

Ingredients:

2 cans drained and rinsed chickpeas
2 tbsp of olive oil
1 paprika teaspoon
1 teaspoon of salt

Directions:

Preheat the oven to 400 degrees Fahrenheit (200 degrees Celsius).

Using a paper towel, pat the chickpeas dry.

Toss the chickpeas in a bowl with the olive oil, paprika, and salt.

On a baking sheet, spread the chickpeas in a single layer.

Bake for 30-40 minutes, or until the bacon is crispy.

Nutritional data (per serving):

186 calories

Fat: 7g
23g carbohydrate
6g fiber
8g protein

Kale Chips with Sea Salt

This snack is a fantastic way to consume kale. Baking kale makes it crispy and crunchy, and seasoning it with sea salt adds a delicious taste.

Time allotted: 25 minutes

2 servings

Ingredients:

4 cups kale leaves, ripped into bite-sized pieces

1 tablespoon extra virgin olive oil

1 teaspoon of sea salt

Preheat the oven to 350 degrees Fahrenheit (175 degrees Celsius).

Toss the kale in a bowl with the olive oil and sea salt.

On a baking sheet, arrange the kale in a single layer.

Bake for 15-20 minutes, or until the bacon is crispy.

Nutritional data (per serving):
81 calories
Fat: 5g
8g carbohydrate
2g fiber
4g protein

Strawberries sliced in Greek yogurt

This sweet and creamy nibble. Greek yogurt has protein and probiotics, while strawberries include vitamin C and antioxidants.
Time allotted: 5 minutes
1 serving size

Ingredients:

1/2 cup plain Greek yogurt
1/2 cup strawberries, sliced
Strawberries should be sliced.
Serve with Greek yogurt.

Nutritional data (per serving):

99 calories
Fat: 0g
12g carbohydrate
2g fiber
12g protein

Slices of turkey with cheese and tomato

This snack is ideal for individuals who want something delicious and satisfying. Protein is provided by the turkey, while taste and nutrients are provided by the cheese and tomato.

Time allotted: 5 minutes

1 serving size

Ingredients:

3 slices turkey

1 cheese slice

1 chopped small tomato

Directions:

Layer the turkey, cheese, and tomato slices in a single layer.

Roll up your sleeves and enjoy.

Nutritional data (per serving):

190 calories

Fat: 9g

5g carbohydrate

1g fiber

22g protein

Sea salt roasted edamame

This snack is a delicious way to eat edamame. Edamame becomes crispy and crunchy after roasting, and sea salt provides a delicious taste.

Time allotted: 30 minutes
Servings per recipe: 4

Ingredients:

2 cups thawed frozen edamame
1 tablespoon extra virgin olive oil
1 teaspoon of sea salt

Directions:

Preheat the oven to 375 degrees Fahrenheit (190 degrees Celsius).

Toss the edamame with the olive oil and sea salt to taste.

On a baking sheet, spread the edamame in a single layer.

Bake for 20-25 minutes, or until the bacon is crispy.

Nutritional data (per serving):

95 calories
Fat: 5g
5g carbohydrate

3g fiber
8g protein

Dark chocolate with cranberries and almonds

This snack is a sweet and filling delight. Antioxidants are provided by dark chocolate, while crunch and taste are provided by almonds and cranberries.
Time allotted: 5 minutes
1 serving size

Ingredients:
1/4 cup dark chocolate chips
a quarter cup almonds
a quarter cup dried cranberries
Melt the dark chocolate chips in the microwave or over a double boiler.
Melt the chocolate and stir in the almonds and cranberries.
Place the mixture on a baking sheet lined with parchment paper.
Freeze for 10-15 minutes, or until the mixture is solid.
Cut into pieces and serve.

Nutritional data (per serving):
238 calories
Fat: 14g
27g carbohydrate
4g fiber
4g protein

Made in United States
Troutdale, OR
07/03/2023

10961869R00046